The First 5

by

J. Mclaurin

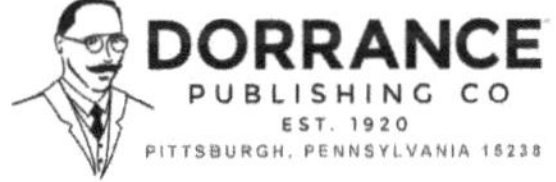

The contents of this work, including, but not limited to, the accuracy of events, people, and places depicted; opinions expressed; permission to use previously published materials included; and any advice given or actions advocated are solely the responsibility of the author, who assumes all liability for said work and indemnifies the publisher against any claims stemming from publication of the work.

Dorrance Publishing Co
585 Alpha Drive
Pittsburgh, PA 15238
Visit our website at www.dorrancebookstore.com

ISBN: 979-8-88683-307-2
eISBN: 979-8-88683-700-1

Table of Contents

This book is dedicated to my beautiful black princess
Azari Mclaurin

The Master Reset Reflections

Since writing *Master Reset* some wonderful things have happened in my life and some not so nice things took place as well. I received some amazing feedback from my book and some amazing fans who loved my work. There have been tons of supporters encouraging me to keep writing and keep telling my story. More importantly, I had individuals encouraging me to keep telling it like it is, spreading knowledge about things in the medical world that people won't share. No one is willing to put their business out there to educate hundreds of others. I wanted to be a blessing to others by sharing my story so that they would know how to handle any medical adversity. My book opened doors for countless interviews and new and meaningful relationships. I was booked and busy, even though we were in a global pandemic, everyone wanted a piece of me, and I appreciated being wanted.

My first book tapped into every emotion one could have and I felt accomplished because that is what I wanted it to do. I was turning my pain into purpose and the fact that people could relate made me smile with glee. All from my home, which at one point made me very depressed, I started a new career as an author. My first manuscript landed me my first book contract; I never even thought my writings were good. Taking full advantage of my God-given talent, *Master Reset* put me in different circles than I was accustomed to. I was now networking with people who had skills I wished to acquire. Things were looking up for me due to the success of my first book and my health appeared to be well managed. I started working out in the gym, even had me a trainer. I started an online business selling sportswear apparel and a young woman that I met, who is now my friend, started inviting me to be a guest on her podcast called *The Muzzle Is Off Podcast*. We met at my book release engagement; she was the first person to interview me about *Master Reset*.

Months before my book was released, I enrolled in college again at Southern New Hampshire University. I only have two years to complete to get my bachelor's degree, so I figured there was no time like the present. It's still a work in progress. but I am happy to report that I am a presidential student. I have surpassed dean's list status, which I think is awesome given that I have a brain injury. I major in communications, so when my friend blessed me with the opportunity to make appearances on her podcast from time to time, she was ultimately investing in my future. I then began to see my village forming that wasn't necessarily kin. I prayed for kindness amongst my friend group, gentleness in the way my people handled me, and lovers of all things beautiful. All my relationships now resembled that and, more importantly, all of them stood tall on the grounds of inclusivity. If it wasn't for me getting sick, I wouldn't have such amazing people in my life that value me and appreciate my testimony.

This love came from pain and with knowing that fact, I embraced the unknown and made it familiar. I started my own business with no capital, just ambition. I crossed into the honors society fraternity at my university and became the first of many in my family. I didn't exactly expect my blessings to be so grand and bold; I just wanted people to feel me. *Master Reset* sparked a lot of raw emotions in people because it was released during a pandemic, a time where everyone longed for a reset. I wanted a reset on top of my reset because even though I was familiar with being home unable to do anything, I wasn't prepared for more loss. The pandemic was taking people out left and right, at an alarming rate. Due to my own troublesome health the lockdown and limitations were real, but I wasn't expecting to lose Evey.

Evey was my great-grandmother, and she also was my friend. Ever since I obtained my brain injury, she has been by my side cheering me on. She always called me to tell me how proud of me she was, and she expressed how excited she was for my first book. It's very unfortunate that she transitioned during the period when the book was in production. It just seems like sometimes everything or everyone I love on hard I lose. It scares me to think that way. It's almost as if I shouldn't love at all because they're going to leave me. The fact of the matter is I never got to know my maternal grandmother because she passed away the year I was born, so Evey, which was her mother—was grandma to me. The relationships I have with my grandparents are special to me because ever since I was thrust into the senior community by circumstance, they became my friends because of relevancy.

We as people are not strangers to death. It happens every day whether we know it or not. The thing that concerns me the most about death in today's climate, is how close it seems to be around me. Not to sound narcissistic, but being as though I have an underlining health condition, I often entertained the notion that I am next. *Master Reset* opened many new doors for me and bolted shut the revolving doors that serve no purpose. I am well respected and known for my demeanor around my city, but more importantly, I am respected for my hard work and tenacity. The combination of pure honesty and transparency are the key factors that made *Master Reset* a success. Now that I am a published artist, people can google me to find out more if they see fit.

I never thought in a million years I would be able to say to individuals "Google me" and or that so many people wanted my autograph. I am still shocked by the whole experience and without a doubt, I am humbled by it also. I pray I always have butterflies in my stomach when someone asks me for a picture and my autograph. It serves as a reminder to always deliver my best self the first time around. At times I know it can seem as if I can't quite make up my mind career-wise, but I am a man with a lot of hidden talents that I always plan to share with the world. I'm less selfish due to my *Master Reset* and to be of service to people in need, fills me up with joy. I displayed the many layers of myself during my *Master Reset* and there is so much more of me that has yet to be explored.

I have goals that I desire and goals that I've already achieved; having a disability did not stop me. As a matter of fact, my disability made me go harder to prove to myself that I could do anything that I dreamed of doing. *Master Reset* taught me a lot about the strength within me and helped me to connect with so many people. To have positive conversations with other like-minded people afforded me a great learning experience. My body of work was created from a space of transparency and inclusion. I wanted my readers to get that feeling when reading my book without me saying a thing. *Master Reset* was an emotion evoker that addressed various subjects in which one can relate. It is also the very thing that drives me to dream bigger and long to expand my platform.

As I write this novel, I would like to acknowledge that nothing is possible for me without Allah (SWT). My family and my supporters are simply the best, all of whom I celebrated and I appreciate it. What I envision for me soon is becoming a life coach. I managed to get my life back on track with the whole world bearing witness to it, and so I would like to help others achieve the same success within. Everyone is so extremely concerned with a makeover for the external version of themselves, that they fail to realize that if you don't heal internally first, nothing on the outside will matter. I would like to be a part of the solution and conversation in reference to healing. My work is far from over; I'm just getting started. *Master Reset* the book was a blessing for me. I matured as a man and became a businessman. Now that I have the first five under my belt, the sky is the limit.

I need people to understand that everything about *Master Reset* was magical. Releasing a book during a pandemic and all the success that came after its release was epic. I'm sure that if there wasn't a pandemic, I could have done so much more with my first novel. I had plans to make it a documentary series via YouTube with me narrating my story, but God had other plans for the world. I was even offered an opportunity to speak about my book at the rehabilitation hospital where I was a patient. I'm still hopeful that I will be able to give back one day. Besides those blessings, I continue to do my part when it comes to being a humanitarian. I am passionate about giving back to the brain-injury community, and I am highly concerned with mental health issues. I feel it is my mission to be a part of both conversations in my community going forward in life. So now that I've updated you on how I've been since my first novel, *Master Reset*, let's explore the *First 5*.

The First Five

I'm sure everyone knows just how crucial the first forty-eight is, but how many people are familiar with the first five? I know for certain that survivors of major medical complications know what it means. Ever since 2017, when all my trauma took place concerning my brain, I was made aware that there were five years that I had to put in the work to remain alive. The doctors explained that after going through chemotherapy and surviving that destructive chemical, they needed to keep me under heavy observation for the next five years. At any giving time during the observation period, I was told I was susceptible to having a third stroke. I was very afraid because my doctors told me that if I did have another stroke, it would probably kill me. Each stroke hits harder and I already had two, so I did my very best to avoid a third one.

Five years of walking on eggshells, getting to know myself, and introducing myself to the world, again. Most people think they know me because they are familiar with me, but they have no clue. Everything in my life changed and although my outer appearance remained the same, my mind was different. I was tainted by my new reality, a life experience filled with hurt, scars, and misery. I was devasted by this pause on my life and so scared at the same time. I didn't want to do anything wrong or go against my doctors' wishes, which was challenging for me because as most of you know, and if you read my first book *Master Reset*, I almost always did the opposite of what was asked of me. In true Leo fashion, I demanded a say in the decisions regarding my life.

So, yes, you guys, I am a faker! I smiled when I didn't have reason smile because no matter what I've accomplished, the first five was always on my mind. I had to play it safe because I couldn't afford any more tragedy, but what I thought was the conclusion to many things, was only the beginning. The amount of mental anguish I endured and chronic anxiety left me stuck in 2017, the year of *Master Reset*. I did my best to be proactive and make something of this time in which I had to fall back, but nothing stopped me from thinking that any false move I made could end my life. I always remained humbled, but I had no time to bask in my glory; I was still fighting for my life. I knew most people wouldn't understand my troubles and I know most people have no clue that I was still on chemotherapy in pill form every day.

My life has been a movie ever since my ordeal, and I think that people appreciated my bounce back more than I did because they only got half of the picture and it was from their point of view. The only piece of the puzzle most had the pleasure of seeing was what I gave away for free. All they knew was that I was sick, and I survived. I gave people something to believe in, made things look easy. My survivor's story unfortunately catapulted me into an elite group of individuals who seem to continuously get tested time after time by God and blessed by God at the same time. However, I didn't see things that way because I feel we are all blessed if we are breathing. Nothing I was doing was special. I think that notion is off putting because I was living everything I wrote. Nothing I wrote about in my first novel was pretty and yet I smiled in public, brushed most things off as if it was no big deal, and behind closed doors I cried like a baby. My nightly prayer was for strength, courage, and wisdom so that I could be prepared just in case I didn't make it to see five years. My situation was so unpredictable that I prepared myself in all aspects for death.

I came to a point where I wasn't afraid of anything. My reality these last five years groomed me to be heavy on survival mode, losing sleep, sometimes literally like an overnight security guard. Most of the time, I didn't like to speak on my health too much because I did not want to jinx my stability. I wanted to put all my afflictions behind me and reintroduce myself to the wonders of life. I did not choose this life, so of course I never got what I wanted in this situation. My struggles with anxiety and depression got better with time, so my opinion on my illness was no longer negative. Based on my experience, the first five had some pros but mostly cons. Not that I need to explain myself to anyone, but if I ever offended anyone with one of my disappearing acts, I apologize. I was struggling mentally. My pride got the best of me, so my worries were never on display, but they were there, raging at times. The ups and downs of these past five years post-intravenous chemotherapy taught me to speak up for myself and be patient with myself. I owed it to myself to properly reintroduce myself to the world. I witness folks switch up on me and I hate that I had to see that. Close friends turned into enemies because they've been hating. The idea that my personality is too much or too big is very offensive to me, just because individuals are insecure. I've been popular all my life both good and bad, so I am not surprised by the fake nor the hate. The only difference is I no longer feel the need to reduce myself or apologize for being me.

Since signing my publishing deal for my first book, I knew the clock was ticking for me to create more legible art. I appreciate my readers and supporters for receiving my body of work well, but I wasn't finished with the momentum of *Master Reset*. I needed to live a little bit to write an interesting story that makes for a good read. I pull everything I write about from my own experience and, just like my first book, the topics I address are very complex. I write to make myself relatable to others and to share the knowledge I obtained during my experience. If you have followed me on my journey to recovery, then you know that there was always something new being introduced to my list of medical problems. My case is not open and shut. I reside in an open-ended realm. I used to think if I could manage to make it to my fifth year of remission, I would be cured. It was a stretch that, quite frankly, was exaggerated by the physicians. At some point I was waiting for all the weight I lost to return, like they said. Due to the way I was treated throughout my experience, I have little to no trust in doctors.

It has been five years and I'm still sick. I am not better nor am I worse; I'm just present. I've had to fight for my life every single year since 2017, and I've had surgery ever single year. In these past five years, I've had ten surgeries, so when I think I'm progressing and moving on with my life, there is always something pulling me back. I'm constantly reminded of all that happened to me, and I'm tried. I don't want to hurt anymore. No one has ever put me down worse than myself. In my head I would think that my friends or family members view me as the disabled one. Therefore, they were going above and beyond to accommodate me but certainly that wasn't the case. I certainly had to learn the difference between genuine concern and negative criticism. Sometimes they both came in the same form and fashion. I had to identify my triggers and set boundaries during my first five, but first I was forced to address problems in a new location.

No Breaks

I wish I could just breathe for a change, but things keep happening to this body of mine. I'm still waiting to exhale. In these past five years, I've had a total of ten surgeries. Everyone should already be aware of the brain surgery, oral surgery, and the stomach surgery, but seven more occurred since then. I haven't been free for the longest time now but going backwards is something that will never be familiar to me. I am all about progression and elevation but when it comes to matters of the body, I have no choice; it is simply a divine thing. Every single year without fail, I managed to land myself on some doctor's operating table.

I underwent four percutaneous nephrolithotomies, one epididymal cysts removal, and a bilateral hip replacement, totaling everything out to ten operations. None of which I saw coming. It is very true that once your body has been attacked at some point, it is never safe again. I honestly shouldn't be shocked, but every time feels like the first time. I desperately wish and pray for no more surgeries, but I don't have a say. I hate going to my follow-up appointments because all they typically share is bad news. New news is just the same as bad news because it is still something that keeps holding me back. I've done so many positive things since I had my strokes back in 2017, but none of that matters if I must keep revisiting my trauma.

The one-year anniversary came and went for my first book *Master Reset*, and I didn't get a chance to take it all in. Dealing with my health was a full-time job and a part-time job. I didn't have a moment just to smell my flowers; the accolades and praise never amused me. It's not that I'm ungrateful; it just felt like wrong timing for me to do. I had a hard time accepting the idea that I was a blessed man when I was clearly being tested year after year. Allah (SWT) really loves me, and I am grateful and amazed by it. I am not the type of person to ever question God, so I won't, but Lord knows I'm tired. I just want it to be over. Enough is enough when it comes to all these surgeries. I have been sliced opened so many times and my latest procedures left scars as proof of this brutal battle.

The most relevant surgery was my bilateral hip replacements. It truly came as a shock to me. I had my moments of reservation but when I think back on how my trauma is set up, I never was allotted breaks. All my surgeries and all my conditions sort of bled into each other so there were never any breaks. But ironically, the only time I did get a break, is when the doctors put my life on pause. I totally had to abandon my progression and put aside my desires for the sake of my life. Never in a million years did I think at the age of thirty-four, I would need my hips replaced. I mean I wasn't an athlete growing up nor did I sustain a prior injury, so you can imagine the curiosity when this hard truth was discovered. *How did I manage to mess up my hips?* That was my first thought because doctors were telling me initially that it was sciatica.

I was experiencing a great deal of sharp pain to my right side in the earlier months of 2021. I first noticed the pain when I was away on a ski trip with my friends in Pennsylvania. I thought the frigid weather had something to do with the aches and pains, since I am anemic. Prior to 2021, I never experienced this type of pain in my right side before, automatically I thought perhaps me being too busy caused pain to my body and I just needed rest. At this point in my life, it is understood that I am disabled by myself and everyone in my life. So, sleep and rest are very important, and for the most part it solves the majority of the problems associated with my illness.

However, this time sleep or rest didn't work. Initially, it was hit and miss—the pain would come but not stay. No amount of stretching worked, but after the ski trip with my friends, I went on another group trip to Miami with another group of friends. The trip was fabulous but without fail the pain attacks started happening again. This time the pain came with blood in my urine. It freaked me out, but I vowed to address this matter once I returned to New Jersey. In a matter of a month things progressed with this issue, the first trip was in March and the second trip was in April. After the trip to Miami and I was back home, the pain grew more intense, and never ever went away again.

I literally began falling all throughout my home, which indicated I was getting weaker. By the time we entered the month of July, I could no longer walk. The doctors insisted it was sciatica at first, but they soon had to rethink that theory when I was found passed out in my home. One day in July, I was home alone, and I couldn't stand the pain, literally and figuratively. I called my mom who was at work and told her I was calling 9-1-1 because I felt bad. I normally wouldn't want to go to the ER because the world was struggling badly with COVID. I was informed prior to this new hurt by my doctors to stay clear of the hospital because I am a high-risk person, so you know the pain had to be bad if I called 9-1-1. When I called the authorities, they instructed me to crawl downstairs to open my front door so they would have easy access to me. I attempted to follow the operator's instructions and successfully made it downstairs in my house by way of crawling. I managed to stand up to unlock the door and screen door to my house.

In my attempt to have both doors opened, I collapsed due to the pain. I was discovered by an Amazon worker who was delivering a package. He was so scared for me that he stayed with me, and he called the ambulance, not knowing I already called 9-1-1 for help. I truly appreciated this stranger who was kind enough to assist me in my time of need, even though it wasn't his job. He only had to stay briefly, however, because my aunt who lives next door had returned home from work. I passed out, but I was conscious, so when my aunt went to pick me up, I advised her not to touch me, simply because I was hurting so bad. The ambulance came shortly after and got me up and assisted me with walking to the ambulance truck. I wouldn't necessarily call what I was doing walking. It was more like I was limping and the EMT workers were dragging me with their arm strength.

The ambulance ride was a bit rocky. I had to share an ambulance with two other people, a woman, and her daughter. Keep in mind COVID was raging, so you know I was paranoid on top of being in a lot of pain. We eventually arrived at University Hospital where I was accosted by a sea of questions but nothing truly in depth. Everything appeared to be smoke and mirrors, and they seemed to be very quick to diagnose me so that they could get me out of there. I was under the impression that my issue really wasn't that serious because they surely didn't investigate further. I was sent home the same night with the same pain and a diagnosis of sciatica, no pain medication just instructions on how to stretch. It came as a shocker when shortly after being diagnosed with sciatica, I was told things were worse than I could imagine. However, the doctor who informed me of this life-altering news didn't seem surprised.

A few weeks after my emergency room visit, I had a follow-up visit with my rheumatologist. My rheumatologist administered my chemotherapy, so he has been in the picture ever since 2017. Going to see him was completely un-related to "sciatica." The visit was a routine follow-up appointment and at this point everything was a struggle. I couldn't walk, couldn't drive, and the pain seemed to be increasing instead of decreasing since my ER visit. I went from a wheelchair to a walker to a cane and eventually began walking independently, but of course, because of this new pain that affected my mobility, I was back walking with the walker. The turnaround in my health made my doctor curious enough to ask about what I was feeling. In my head, I was thinking this issue had nothing to do with him and his expertise, but I continued to explain my pain anyways. At the end of my visit, he ordered me to go get an X-ray done immediately, I thought that was weird, but I did the X-ray that very same day. Within the two hours it took for me to get home that very same doctor called me with some devastating news. It turned out I now have a new condition called Avascular Necrosis and I needed to undergo bilateral hip surgery.

Incurable

As you can see, I literally can't catch a break, now all of a sudden, I have avascular necrosis. I was stunned to find out that I have a new condition and the solution was hip replacement surgery, but the worst part of it all—I was stuck with this condition. To my knowledge it is incurable, and it is brought on by the overuse of steroids. Now, I am the type of patient who follows the doctor's orders, and I am also very inquisitive, however, I was trying to figure out when was I given steroids. I thought I knew all that happened to me, and I thought it was far behind me, sadly it was not. My past scarred me badly, and honestly, I didn't want to revisit it, but to find out how this ordeal came to be, I had to take this fright-fest roller coaster into my past.

Baffled but this horrible news, the first person I inquired information from was my doctor who discovered the problem. It was a bit strange that he knew where to look. Not only did he know where to look, he automatically sent me a script in the mail for an orthopedic surgeon. I didn't fully process this new information and the name of it, so to get the script in the mail a few days later was surprising. The call to this doctor was a bit strange. He acted as if this was common for a person that is thirty-four years old to need new hips. He further explained certain treatments that I received four years ago were the reason why my hips were now corroded. How was that even possible? When was the doctor going to say or do something to intercept this disease?

Avascular necrosis is the death of bone tissue due to a lack of blood supply. Also known as osteonecrosis and can be caused by long-term steroid use and drinking too much. I was not the drinker post-trauma due to my illness, so the drinking cause did not pertain to me. When trying to put the pieces together, I was often confused. I reached back out to the doctor who discovered the issue and asked him, "Who did this to me?" I was violated and I wanted to know who did this to me. He gave me a wild goose chase from hell. I began to wonder what is it that he's trying to hide. He stated that with me having so many doctors on my roster and so many treatments, who's to say who did this to me. I began doing my own investigation because he was of no help. I began pulling all my medical records from each hospital I'd ever stayed in. It was easy to get my records but very difficult to understand them because doctors talk in code and the medical terms weren't familiar to me.

Once again, I had to rely on the doctor who discovered the disease to help me better understand certain terms from an establishment not affiliated with the hospital where he works. In the midst of trying to find out who did this to me, I was also setting up an appointment to see a hip surgeon to discuss my options. It seems like the discovery doctor was convinced the previous hospital caused me to have avascular necrosis, but none of the paperwork supported his claim. I went to see the surgeon who could potentially work on my hips. This is when things got a bit interesting. The first surgeon I went to go see took images of my hips, which confirmed that they indeed needed to be replaced. When asked how I sustained this injury, I couldn't explain how I got this injury because I didn't know. Skimming through all my medical records didn't provide me any answers so I had to reach back out to the doctor who discovered it.

To my surprise he had the answers, when I called, I told him I needed black and white proof to give to the surgeon. He mailed me the printout with highlighted areas indicating steroid usage and this whole time the person I was searching for was him. He knew where to look when I was suffering in pain, he sent the referral via the mail ASAP for surgery, and he provided the evidence that was requested by the orthopedic surgeon as proof that steroids did this to me. I was insulted because up until that moment, that doctor was good to me. I believe that his mistake was that he wasn't on top of things but by no means do I feel like he was moving in malice. He treated me and my condition like the average patient scenario and nothing about me or my condition is ordinary. The very treatment the doctor performed on me to save my life is the very same treatment that caused me to now have avascular necrosis.

Thinking back on it now, I believe he sent me the referral in the mail so fast because he wanted to cover his tracks. He failed me as physician. I had no knowledge of steroid usage and neither did my family. He failed to properly notify me and my family about what the treatment entailed and most importantly its side effects. It seemed to me that I was the only one left in the dark and the only one suffering due to negligence or incompetence. There was a time when I thought I was in the clear. I mean I knew the conditions that I had were incurable, but I thought they were at least sustained. My first novel, *Master Reset*, spoke to my warm embrace and acceptance of my new normal. I had to learn the new me and my new body since the old me was never ever found and was presumed deceased.

I learned how to work with the right side of my body even though it has been numb for five years. I changed my diet to promote healthy eating since studies have shown that most of the food we grew up on is the cause of illnesses that most people face today. I was very proactive in my growth as a man but more importantly as a survivor. Sickness seemed to still follow me. I now have two new titanium robotic hips that have altered my life, all due to avascular necrosis. I am undergoing another master reset that I am calling "A Change of Plans." I expected things to go one way, but God clearly had other plans for me. The surgeries were painful, each experience healed differently, and they weren't done at the same time. I had my first one done on September 16, 2021, and the second surgery was completed on January 3, 2021. They both left me with horrible scars on my thighs, and a horrible thought on my mind. I suffered for so long I can't tell you which procedure I had over the years I deemed to be the worst. I have been at war with myself for five years, so even the pandemic didn't move me.

Everything I've been through should have me hating life by now, but I refuse because even when I'm down, I'm never out. All my conditions don't make me sad nor ashamed. They just let me know how favored I am, although they are incurable. When the enemy decides to attack, which is sickness, I suit up in my armor gear and prepare the others because I am about to give it a fight of my life. All I know how to do is be strong. My mother raised me that way. I walk around now with hips that cost $80,000 and insurance doesn't cover the entire bill, so one of these doctors has some explaining to do. Going forward in the midst of this situation, I decided to defeat another struggle of mine. It just so happened to be next on my agenda. I guess you can say my birthday came early because while still very much in chromic pain, I decided to quit smoking for good. I started off with the patches but relapsed at my convenience.

When it was made clear that I must stop to have my procedures, I realized that playtime was over. I had to grow up in that very moment and, I knew for all the good things I was doing to my body, that one negative action made the good things null and void. The ultimatum forced me to quit smoking and I never looked back, but at first it was a challenge. It became a test that challenged discipline and checked my ego. I had no room to play games. It was a matter of life or death, and I wanted to win.

Cigarettes

I've been smoking cigarettes since I was nineteen years old, not once did I find this habit to be a problem. I was an adult when I made the decision to smoke, and besides, at the time, both my parents smoked. In my house it was viewed as a norm. And if anything, I was afraid to do it around them because I never wanted to be disrespectful or disappoint them. I thought it relieved stress and made up for a hectic schedule, so I saw no problem with it. When it came to odor or the look of all, I quite frankly didn't feel it applied to me. I was one of those fashionable adults that was popular all my life, so I set the trends; I never followed any of them.

However, I later discovered that I was following my parent's footsteps and so many adults before me who viewed cigarettes as a way out. Even with that knowledge, I continued to smoke. I started off at first with the cowboy cigarettes, Marlboros. Everyone clowned me for my choice in cigarettes. I am a black man, so most people stated that they felt I should be smoking Newport's, but there is no manual that instructed me on the dos and don'ts of smoking. The whole idea of smoking is a bad idea wrapped in good intentions. I smoke to relieve me of stress and I'm fully aware that there are other means to doing such things, but I like what I like. If I am being honest with myself, which I usually am, I don't think I will ever be completely free from cigarettes.

I consider myself a part-time smoker now because although I have made great strides and am not currently smoking, the urge is still there. To say I'm not a smoker and yet still back-door smoke is emotional and mental abuse. It suggests that I am pretending to be free of the habit for society's sake, and that I am not a human who will make mistakes. In return I don't feel the need to place unrealistic and ridiculous standards on myself, and when or if ever I fall off the wagon, I will not assume the position of my very own bully. I am for sure not interested in causing harm to myself mentally. After all my own body is constantly trying to end me. I guess withstanding the facts that my body is trying to ruin me, I can't possibly consider smoking the worst thing in the world. However, the underlining issues for me smoking must be addressed.

Since I am an individual who has been granted a master reset, who also is forever on a healing safari, I need answers. To find them I had to look inward. Cigarettes weren't the cause of my medical trauma, but I'm pretty sure it didn't make things any better. Cigarettes are not the air that I breathe nor the food I eat for nourishment, so I wonder why they have such a strong hold on me. I was nineteen years old when I started smoking cigarettes, so I had to retrace sixteen years of old footsteps to discover where things went wrong. It was much deeper than just liberty and fun that caused me to smoke. Had it been simply that, I would've quit. Per the way I operate, I put my efforts and energy into finding out about me and what were my triggers sixteen years ago. I needed to know specifics. I reached deep down in my unconscious and blew dust off the old books of mine, to recall scenarios and situations that caused me to smoke in that moment. I wanted to know did my stress have a name or a gender. I wondered was it constant and frequent, I wanted to be able to identify it when I was under a great deal of stress in any moment.

I began incorporating mediation into my daily routine, and to think of it, if my hips didn't rot out, I would have never considered quitting cigarettes, which led me on a journey to discover my triggers. As old as I am, you would think I knew my triggers, but I seriously did not. All my life I assumed my attitude was holding me back or it was the fact that I had tremendous pride, but it clearly was none of that. I wish it was that simple to explain, but I slowly started to notice that everything that I was doing at any giving moment was brought on by an experience. I do what I do now because of something I experienced in my past and my brain stored the information and now it is using it as my trigger, unconsciously. I needed to be able to pinpoint the moments in my life that caused me pain and reflect on the negative experiences in my past, so that I could have peace.

I deserved to be happy, but I have yet to be familiar with that feeling. I think for the last five years, I've been playing it safe out of fear that things medically would get worse and personally out of fear that too much of anything could overwhelm me. Smoking provided relief when my world got crazy, even if it only lasted few minutes. I would escape life a few moments (smoke break) and then come back to my reality prepared to fight some more. I am not condoning something that is of poor health and of poor choice, I am simply telling my truth. I don't judge, so I would appreciate if folks didn't do it to me because I am human just like the rest of the people in the world. What is life without mistakes? And where are the people who've never made any? I never asked to be this beacon of strength or perfection. All I ever wanted was to just be myself. I seemed to have mastered not smoking, at least on a full-time spectrum, so if I can do it, anyone can.

If you feel you need to stop smoking, then I think you should try. An addict of any sort is an addict of sorts. Take things day by day like I do, and guess what? If you fall short, it is okay. You can be cigarette-free for six-plus months and if for some reason you decide to smoke again but not constantly, you are okay in my eyes. Dust yourself off and try again.

Success is not the destination, it is the journey. I share my story to make other people aware that they are not alone. Being honest with yourself is key and being less critical of yourself decreases stress. If you are a person searching for balance in your life, then you will understand the work that I've done to sort out my triggers. There is not one moment in our past that we can do over, but we have a moral obligation to ourselves to acknowledge every impactful moment in the name of healing. It is important to acknowledge the hurt or what we have seen so that we never have to experience an event like that again. To promote and increase harmony, one must invest in themselves and begin the work on the internal them.

I don't know if I am going stay smoke-free for the rest of my life, though that is the plan. I purposely choose not to harp on that thought. I'd just show up and make the effort every single day. I think the beauty in my experience as a smoker is that it is a piece of my puzzle that is needed to render a complete picture of myself. It has brought me closer to being somewhat whole again and I have gained peace with many situations since I decided to quit. If I have a cigarette today or tomorrow, it is okay to because not too long ago, I was smoking a pack a day. People see me and can't believe me when I express, "I am a smoker." My skin, teeth, nor lips suggest this notion. I guess I have great genes. I never smelled like it because I was very conscientious of my appearance given the circumstances. When my vice seemed at some point to be out of control and was bad for my health, I knew playtime was over. I had to kill the monster and I started damage control by first cutting off its head, and when doing so, I had to execute it perfectly so that it would not return.

I found it resourceful to dive deeper into my past and present to recognize triggers and avoid them. The more I learned about myself and my sensitivity sensors, the more successful I became in beating this awful habit. So, now that the smoke has cleared and the attempt has been initiated to live a smoke-free life, let me describe my trigger awareness journey.

Triggers

Discovering my triggers was not an easy feat. Let's be honest. Who wants to admit any form of weakness, at least that's what it seems like? From the little bit of memory that remains in my unconscious after the strokes, I don't recall being as sensitive. To me sensitivity does not equate to synthetics, meaning just because you are sensitive does not mean your skin isn't tough. In fact, the strongest and toughest person tends to be the most sensitive one of them all. The thing is, they are stellar at concealing and hiding it and would rather display anger instead. So here we go with the angry black man or woman narrative. If only we were properly taught healthy communication skills. Us as people have been constipated with trauma for the longest and I wasn't willing to be just another statistic. It was important for me to discover my triggers because I didn't want to spark another stroke by ignoring them.

I think all my life up until now I wasn't so self-aware and lived life unbothered. It wasn't until I got sick that I noticed that certain treatments and or behaviors triggered me, both from other people and myself. Things had to change for the betterment of me and I was prepared to do whatever it required. During this process I lost people that I thought would be in my life forever, but unfortunately, they were only in my life for a chapter not the entire book. A hard truth and painful reality, but I desired peace and anyone or anything standing in my way had to be removed. I discovered through this process of elimination that I was extremely tolerable and not sensitive at all. I allowed people to be who they wanted to be in my life, and I never said a word. I couldn't change them. I could only change their access to me, yet I just took whatever they gave me for years

I had everyone's back but my own, putting the needs of others before mine, and that mentality almost killed me. I internalized a lot and although I was being mistreated, I never changed my position and folded on the person I vowed to always be there for. I grew to understand I allowed the mishandling of me for years and that was also a trigger. For all the things I've done for others and how much I gave to others, I couldn't believe they would take advantage of me and do me so wrong. I had to learn to appreciate myself more and cut off the selfish individuals. So, the first trigger I identified and addressed was selfish people. I no longer felt bad when I said no, and I no longer felt like it was my call of duty to have another's back when it wasn't reciprocated. I simply would wish them the best and continue being around people who poured into me, like I poured into them.

Please understand that I am fully aware that no one is going to leave this world unscathed, we all go through trials and tribulations, so I can't begin to tell you I knew what the other person must've been going through internally. I don't blame anyone; some people simply didn't have the tools necessary to love or feel. It took me to get sick to notice I was getting the short end of the stick. To blame anyone for things getting out of hand other than myself, would be me giving the other party too much credit. The beauty in being an honest and fair person is that I get to see things from both perspectives. It allows room for me to forgive the other person and more importantly forgive myself; you move on quicker in my opinion and surrender to the peace you've made. I never knew I also had abandonment issues until now, again I let people be who they wanted to in my life, even if I seem to disagree.

I think most of my readers are wondering about my other parent. I speak so highly of my mom and say nothing about my dad. The reason being is because I don't truly know him. My father and mother were married, and he is the dad to me and all my siblings, and yes, he was around. It's sad that I never get chances to bond with the man I greatly resemble—according to public opinion. In my opinion it is him who stops that from happening by way of mistreatment. Who I am today, which is a proud black gay man, is who he assumed I would be back then, when I was kid. My identity and preference didn't come into play until I was eighteen years of age but by then I had already been written off in my opinion. For the record I love him for the sake that he is my father and as I write about him, I automatically feel the need to protect him, even if it kills me. As a matter of fact, it almost did, if only he knew all the things I have done just for his approval.

Sometimes I wish I could un-love him because maybe it wouldn't hurt me so bad, especially when it appears he don't care. Ever since I was a younger adult, I took on jobs and roles in life that demonstrated leadership and hyper-masculinity. At times I may have been uncomfortable, but I took the job regardless only to make him proud. I wanted him to see that I was decent, and I was nothing like he thought I would be. I broke my neck to satisfy that man because I was raised by him and my mom very well. Respect was instilled in me since I was a little boy. I will be forever grateful that my parents introduced me and my brothers to Islam but other than that, he didn't handle me correctly. Before anyone can say my mother planted a seed, folks must consider what I've witnessed with my own eyes. The trauma replays in my mind so many times, but the cycle of mental abuse has concluded. It took me to get sick to see that my daddy issues chapter needed to end. For many years I took on responsibilities and jobs that were very stressful just to prove to him that I am a man. I punished myself by neglecting my own health, just to prove to him that I was hard too and not all soft.

Soft by society's standards meant you were weak and less of a man, so everything that I possessed I attempted to work it out of me. The point is that I made myself ill and have since been diagnosed with a brain injury, a hard and ugly truth. The mental abuse was so bad that once I became sick, I thought that meant I would get more attention from him. In my sick and twisted mind I thought he would be there for me finally and I would finally get my turn. For once I thought the focus would be on me after all I endured with medical trauma. All I ever wanted was for my father to see me and love me, I am his first-born, my birth made him a dad. Here I am fighting for my life and my father is nowhere to be found. Year after year, surgery after surgery and it appeared that he could care less. I went through this traumatic battle without his attention or presence. I'd finally had enough. I learned he is never going to be the dad I want him to be for me and I also realized that although I want him in my life that I don't need him. I am my own man now and I can't take anyone's disrespect, not even if it's my father.

I can't speak to his remorse or his feelings because we've never had a man-to-man conversation, I was never allowed to express myself around him. In my healing journey I discovered my worth and the fact that I had to cut off all sources who drained me of my peace, love, and energy. I needed to be free of all my triggers and I am an honest man who can admit my dad was a huge trigger. I am also aware that I will never totally be free of him because we are kin, but I am free of his hold on me. I will always respect him, but my love and heart are too pure to be trampled over or to be thrown away like yesterday's trash, so I decided to keep it moving. I realized that trying to be the ultimate perfectionist almost killed me. My heart was in the right place at the time, but now I know the errors in my ways.

Some may think or say it's too late to have realized these major triggers, but I beg the differ, because had I not identified that I am a grown man with both little-boy trauma and daddy issues, I think I wouldn't be sane today. These sorts of things eat away at you and no matter how old you get or are, the pain your younger self endured will still plague you. It will haunt you and suck the life out of you and you wouldn't have a clue as to why. Sometimes the why isn't always found or has a clear and direct contact, but it's worth diving into. I say that because maybe along that journey you may perhaps get some sort of closure. I may not ever get that conversation with my father, but I have made peace with it. That is not to suggest that I am excusing his behavior. It just means I'm learning to do the best with what I got.

At some point as I was maturing, I realized my parents weren't superman and superwoman; they were human just like myself. They are just a man and a woman, once I understood that concept, I became less critical of them. I've made my share of mistakes so who am I to crucify my father. Yes, of course I would like more of him, and sure I would have liked for him to show up for me, but that's not what we are dealing with here. Parents do their best and sometimes their best isn't good enough, but all things go, so we must move on to grow. To be the person we envisioned ourselves to be, we must let go of our past trauma because that just might be the one thing that is stopping us from going to the next level in our lives. The triggers mentioned in this chapter are just a few from a chapter in my life, there are so many others, and some are eternal.

Since our help doesn't come from outside of us, there are certain actions and behaviors that we do unconsciously that are harmful to the person we are today. We solicit negative things into our lives by what we tolerate in our world. In the moment, if our mind does not respond negatively, we assume it's what we need, but once things become incessant our mind throws in a red flag. At that moment the body is alerted, and we began to differentiate the needs from the wants. The first step is realizing your triggers and setting boundaries so that you could have peace in your reality.

Still Growing Up

Throughout the voyage I selected to go on, I discovered a lot of things about myself that I never bothered to ever explore. All my life I compartmentalize every aspect of my being, and prioritized each moment from least to favorite, based on what I thought was important. The war began when I never returned to address the least. I had a closet filled with bodies that never received the proper burial. I would pile them up to the point where they all overlapped, and it wasn't until I got stricken with an illness that I found all of those remains. I had tons of skeletons and each body represented a piece of me that I left behind to die. The number of bodies that I accumulated could no longer be contained, therefore I had no choice but to identify each body. I was forced to grow up and face the naked truth.

The truth that no one knew, not even me, the task seemed like torture at first, but I gradually adjusted and embraced the transformation. This change of plans challenged everything I grew to be okay with from my traumatic 2017. Just when I thought I knew all that I needed to know about my body and mind, the doctors piled on more complications I had to consider. I had to stop my progression and do research about new conditions that are now a part of my narrative. Learning that the stop of medication can lead to me becoming brain dead, that alone had me shook. For the rest of my life, I will be uncomfortable, especially with my new artificial hips. somehow doctors want me to perhaps smile through this life experience. I never found it amusing and I never will. Me surviving is simply not enough. While growing up in this experience, I had to learn how to have a mean poker face.

The carpet didn't match the drapes in this instance, so the fact that I am afflicted with so much pain, my books do me no justice. I had to learn this new body filled with so may surgical scars that I hate and more conditions than an entire football team. Most people would faint or die if they were made to endure just one of my surgeries. Like always I use my life experience as a tool to help others, so I am an open book. My doors are always open as well and I will always be one phone call away. I never want another person to go through what I had to go through and if someone was dealt similar cards, I want them to know they are not alone. I will hold their hand every step of the way because the road ahead of them is dark and lonely. I wish I had someone who was familiar with this level of pain there to support me and since I didn't, I vow to stand by another in need. I am placed in the category as a martyr nowadays, but I will never see myself as the world sees a person like me. Nothing that I've done to me is worthy of a Nobel Peace Prize. I'm simply just being myself.

The chain of events in my life shaped and molded that man I am today. From the bullying to the countless fights, to the countless times I felt let down or disappointed, they all make me who I am. My life has been somewhat filled with turbulence at times, but whose life hasn't? That mere fact is what forbids me from looking at myself and my situation as a miraculous phenomenon. I am not a hero; I am just Jamal, and whatever comes with being me, I embrace wholeheartedly. I have come to learn that just when I thought I knew all I needed to know about being an adult, there was twice as much stuff I didn't know about being an adult. It took for me to be stripped of everything that I was fond of in my life, to truly explore what it really means to be "grown." I had the responsible, money-making part down to a science, but in caring for one's heart and mind, I faltered.

Two essential components that should never be excused at any time in someone's life, I dismissed with ease. I never considered how crucial they were until mine were tampered with; I wasn't prepared for the troubles that came with this form of neglect. I spent countless hours researching all the diseases that have become me and at some point, took over me. The only factors I was ever truly concerned with in the beginning were the how's and the why's. I knew for sure who was the topic of discussion, and I knew when it all took place, but no one was ever able to explain to me why all this happened to me, and how did this all occur in my life. Things took their own shape and had their way with my body, completely opposite of what I envisioned for my life. Every human has their breaking point, but I can honestly say, although I was broken, I never desired a break. I was content with the constant rolling of this train because I was assured by God that the victory was mine.

I learned to rely on faith and not to be so hard on myself. I made it my daily practice to begin my day with gratitude. I learned to love my life even on the days that I hated my body. Even when my days seemed dark, lonely, and cold, I was still grateful. I know my suffering has not been in vain and I know one day I will rejoice and sing. I find myself growing little by little each day. That is what makes me feel alive. My new lease on life began in my mind first and my body began practicing the same philosophy. This was not a one-shot deal, I had to become the exercise in order to master it. Every day going forward in my life, I must have a talk with myself in effort to keep me mentally in check. There is freedom in healing from past trauma. The concept can be brutal, but it is also eye-opening. You can potentially discover what you have stored in your unconscious that no longer serves you.

Indeed, I am the same man with somewhat the same appearance. People can't see the tiny stretch marks I've gained throughout this grow-up transition. I had to expand and grow so much to the point in my mind I was an overweight man who wore a size 40w pants. In reality, of course, I was not that large, but my mind was on the verge of exploding with knowledge. I had grown in ways that I didn't think were possible given my age, and I gained a better understanding of what was taking place in my medical file. Most importantly I came to terms with the fact that doctors sometimes can be your worst asset. You may think they are on the same page as you, but somehow, they still manage to screw you over. The overall objective should be to make you better not string you along and cause future problems for you that you yourself can't foresee. Doctors have a way with words and will use you like a guinea pig for a trial they strongly believe may be the next break in medicine. I've learned to be my own doctor, nurse, and therapist because to medical personnel you are just a cash cow. I can't express enough how much my family and I put our trust in doctors because we assumed they knew more, but they did not.

I grew. I've learned and with God's permission I will grow some more. I appreciate the man I am, flaws and all, and I am excited by thoughts of the man I will be, and I am less concerned about the man I used to be. I grew into that frame of mind. I am destined for greatness; I've always been great, I just forgot who I was along the way. On several attempts, many people tried to remind me of that notion but until God testifies on behalf of your greatness, you may never know. I am the choosing one for the proof is out there in the universe. It's out there for everyone to see. I share me furthermore with the world so that people can understand and see that even when you get knocked down hard, you must always pick yourself up and try life again. If you are ever conflicted or afflicted with something and you are afraid to voice your concern, speak to someone you trust and ask for help. I am aware that pride gets the best of all of us, but we must allow ourselves the time to be human and get the help we need. The biggest takeaway for me still growing up is that I learned that vulnerability is strength. It is me saying I had this issue that is bigger than me and I need help fighting this demon.

I am no longer afraid or worried about judgment. I am more concerned that If I don't get the proper help with my demon, I will become the demon. I vowed to choose me today and every day. My mental, physical, and spiritual health are far more important than my ego. I don't care what it takes, I just want to be okay. The first five has been a roller coaster and this part of the ride I am grateful to reflect on. Thank you to everyone who joined me on this ride. The growth let me know God was not done with me, that he was tired of seeing me cry. I take life for what it is—the good, the bad, and the ugly. I celebrate all things big and small for I know the dark side, but I refused to claim that as my residence. Cheers to me and cheers to all for standing when they had the option to sit, and salute to all the soldiers who are not here to do either.

There are all countless things we face daily and yet we never give up. You don't need to be faced with medical problems to relate to me or my story; being human is enough to comprehend that we may share likeness. Triumph is triumph and victory is victory. As people we are quick to celebrate others and not ourselves and I don't blame anyone. We all have been indoctrinated. Generation after generation of people being told to be proud of yourself is a bad thing, you must stay humble. Life is hard enough by itself and can throw you all sorts of curve balls, so to have people reduce your winnings is traumatizing. The kind of behavior that we have been tolerating for years is the same reason why we look at each other as enemies instead of brothers and sisters. We have a duty to make the world better for our children by putting an end to this sort of behavior.

We must deprogram ourselves just to reprogram ourselves in the correct format. This process will not happen overnight. It takes willingness, but until then, I will celebrate times two, for both me and you.

Celebrating X2

I know most people have no clue what it means to "celebrate times two." I don't blame them because I didn't either until I created the phrase. To celebrate times two is something I started saying only after my trauma. I saw the world different and when speaking to other survivors, our sentiments were the same. It seemed to me that the point of view was different for body-able individuals and disabled people when it comes to the topic of celebration. I know everyone who faced trauma are not disabled, but I am disabled, and this is my perspective. It seems as though today people look at a celebration as something that is a giving, with consideration of the occasion. That is a privilege someone disabled does not have. Every event that they are allowed to attend reminds them that they are still alive. Two parties that consist of humans and yet two separate approaches when it comes to celebrating.

Don't get me wrong. There is not a right or wrong way to celebrate, but a person like me celebrates for the me that died and the me now. If I overindulge, just leave me be, because you may not know all it took for me to still be here. I am happy to see my family and friends enjoying themselves because there were numerous times during these past five years that I thought for sure I was going to die. I enter every event amazed and surprised because I am there to see it with my own two eyes, not in spirit but in the flesh. To dance, to cheer people on, get dressed up, allow me to feel alive. It feels good to feel again when based on my injury I should be cold, "six feet under the ground" cold. That is my truth and my reality, so absolutely I celebrate times two, because I'm going to enjoy this one and only go 'round in this thing called life.

There are no do-overs, so you must make the most of it. When you learn to put yourself first and understand that there is more to life, you, too, will began celebrating times two. Time fly's they say, but the more time spent on this earth you will understand that time is an illusion, so stop counting the years as a badge of honor; stay in the present. Capture every moment, take it all in, the good the bad and the ugly. As a disable black man, I started celebrating everything twice because I didn't think of anything besides my trauma. I thought for sure daily I was not going to be around to celebrate anything, so every chance I get, I do it big. I honestly don't regret a thing, every sloppy drunk moment I own because that is my spirit having fun with my inner demons. Why do you think a drunk mind speaks a sober truth? Here come the negative Nancys and the negative Normans with their two cents about how you should live your life as if we are all the same.

They want you to trust in that same two cents that could never buy them anything. It's safe to say thank God they were not being paid to think. Have your fun because only you know how hard it is to be you, and how all that you've been through shaped and molded you to be the person you are today. Take time to introduce people to the new you because most people only understand change from a physical standpoint. You have grown in ways that the eyes simply can capture, so never crucify others; instead teach them. Take them on a ride as you celebrate times two and pray that one day, they will be able to do it too. They are not the ones that hurt you. It's not as much of their fault as it is yours. I understand completely the contemplation of forgiving others. You weren't allotted the same liberty of just being, so why give them a second chance? You are not their creator, so you can't judge, the forgiveness isn't for them; it is for you. I had a moment in my life where I ran with that same mentality, I thought that was the proper way to operate, but in the end, I suffered mentally. That approach for me did not work; instead I decided to try a little tenderness.

The part that is missing from mankind is the kind part. Often, we give away too much of our energy to what is wrong and not enough to what is right. If you feel like you are not being treated the way you would like to be treated, turn the situation into a teachable moment instead of casting a stone. We all make mistakes and I know at some point we all have a God complex, and we think we can be so cruel to others. The higher power is looking down upon us like "excuse me, who are you?" Once I did my self-work and found a deeper meaning to life, I took all that I've learned and brought it back to my people. I never found satisfaction in being around a group of people that did not know anything, and I knew more, especially the people I say I love. I guess I had to learn all the lessons so that my people can eat off my blessings. I say that with love because it was my people that lifted me up and supported me no matter what. My struggle was not and still is not in vain. I take my victory lap for those who came before me and those who joined me. We made it!

Life has a funny way of humbling us and it is up to us to learn from the lesson. I did not choose to have a brain injury; however, I did decide what I would do with a brain injury. God didn't give up on me, so I was not going to give up just because I have an invisible disability. As I grew, everyone around me was growing. We all now know what it is like to be living with a disability and what it is like to be battling depression. I didn't care if I had to be the catalyst for people in my community just so that they gain more knowledge and understanding. I cared to be free from all the pain, hurt, and the guilt, I discovered that if everyone around me knew my injury thoroughly, they could be an ally to assist me in achieving my goal. Some people wanted the same thing for themselves, so they came on board because they understood where I was coming from.

Celebrating times two in the first five years at first seemed a bit challenging because in the beginning I had nothing to be jovial about. A lot of time initially was spent feeling sorry for myself and getting to know myself again. Eventually, I got tired of the self-hatred and decided to do something to change the narrative. I was never the type of person that fit in any category or box, so fitting the stigma of being the helpless disabled man was never going to happen. Against counsel I exploited my disability to help others; things that I should have kept private I shared anyway. I was sacrificing myself again, but this time I was doing it in a less stressful way. When things were bad for me, I couldn't find anyone who could share the wisdom of tragedy. There weren't any services for people who looked like me and was coming from where I was from, so I created the space. The conversation about our mental health is a conversation that is way overdue.

Throughout these past five years allowed me the opportunity to see how programed we are as people. We are taught celebrating too big means that we are bragging, and that we need lessons on how to be humble. Overachieving is looked at as an insecurity of the sorts and I hate that for us. I created celebrating times two because what most people fail to realize is that before you managed to succeed, you had to lose. The first attempt isn't always successful, but you didn't give up. The very fact that you didn't give up is the reason you've been rewarded with a win. In my case I had a life before my injury and once I was dealt the two strokes, that old Jamal died. I was weak, but I wasn't broken and, more importantly, I did not quit. I had a second chance at life, but this time I wanted it to be meaningful and better than before. My life is not without fault, so sometimes I don't feel my best, but that does not stop me from giving life the best that I got.

The next time you ever consider misjudging a person like me who celebrates times two, remember what they may have endured is far more damaging than what you could ever fathom. You never know what a person has gone through and all they really would need from you is kindness. Society has taught us that there is a certain look to grieving as it is to happiness, but I'm here to challenge that theory. As humans we come in varieties and so does glee. It's up to the individual to decide their preference. The choice is based on comfortability and there is not a right or wrong way to do it. Live life on your terms unapologetically and continue to show up for yourself. I had to learn this mantra the hard way because it didn't come easy for me. Naturally, I always looked at my proudness as something I should be ashamed about. I know now that I was light-years ahead of the world and so as I was healing myself, I felt I owed younger me an apology.

An open letter to young Jamal

Dear Young Jamal,

I'm writing you this letter because I need you to know how much you mean to me and the world. Your life is going to be hard but everything you need will already be inside of you. You are going to open doors for a lot of people, demonstrating to the world that you are here and your voice matters. You are going to love with deep passion, but I want you to be careful of the amount of energy you pour into others. That type of behavior creates the space for enabling and there will come a point in your life when people are going to take advantage of you. You are smart, creative and, most certainly, you a leader. You will spend a great deal of your youth trying to make people see value in you when you don't even see it for yourself first. The strength you possess is divine yet will be tested numerous times. You are going to experience a lot of sadness but will see yourself through it all. Please remember that you did nothing wrong, and everything is not your fault, hold your head high.

The bubbly baby boy who you grew to love will be snatched away from you at four years old. Stepping into the world of schooling you are going to meet some cruel people. It will appear at first as if you don't have any friends, but you will soon understand that it will be a matter of who is a real friend and who is not. The torture you will come to know will carry on all through your elementary years. It's going to cause you to hate yourself. You are going to begin hating your voice, your walk, and the way you look. You are smart, but no one notices that when they are busy making you feel like the scum of the earth. Your heart will become cold, and your feelings will become numb to the tough. You will be robotic in movement, sound, and thought. No matter where you are, you will never feel safe, and the only pain reliever is your mother. Physical altercations are going to become familiar for a person like you.

Even when hurt you still show up in times of adversity. You have a true since of family and community, but there will be those who will forsake you. There will be a lot of awkward moments such as parents not allowing their kids to befriend you and insecure moments around other boys, especially during gym in school. You are going to feel like you don't belong anywhere but in your mother's arms. As you mature, you will have a sense of who you would like to be, even though it will be years before you will gain the strength to live out loud. You will be very popular for both good and bad reasons, but once you find your groove, you will become a champion for people like yourself. Although it wasn't on purpose, you will forge a lane for individuals to just be themselves, you will become the example for many on what it means to regain your power. You will be broken, but you will never give up, everything in your life will make sense in due time. Never being truly satisfied is what will compel you to achieve a lot in your life.

You are going to think it is necessary to be perfect all the time just so that others won't leave you. Just when you start truly loving the young man that you are becoming, a complexity will surface again. At nineteen years old, the idea of homosexuality will come into play, a mindset that you fought so hard to change. Your life's work and mission will be grounded in individuality, but who you lay down with is the only thing people will talk about. You are going to feel like your pursuit of happiness is a luxury and not a God-given right. You are going to feel like you don't deserve to be happy because the world decrees you to death. The world will convince you that the moment you call yourself gay, you can no longer consider yourself a man. You are going to have to find yourself in gay culture too because, even there, you are not going to fit in. Years of oppression are going to convince you that it's you against the world. The formation of the wall that you built will be created with hurt, sadness, and confusion, and hard to tear down.

You are always going to wonder why people hate you so much and you are going to feel like you have missed out on being a kid. You are aged by trauma and in those moments, you are going feel like this is the worst thing that can happen to a person. Fashion and artistry are where you will soar, but you will feel like something is missing. Self-doubt will force you to cancel yourself out of the love department because you feel like no one will ever love you. You figured you must make nice with women because the men will not welcome you in their fraternity. The only males that are willing to be all-inclusive with you are your brothers. They love you the way you are for how you are is all they've ever known. Brokenhearted and all, you will still manage to gather the will and skills to survive in this cruel and cold world.

I can promise you, little Jamal, that you are going to be larger than life one day. People are going to have to take a number in reference to hanging out with you. Contrary to all the days you cried asking God to please make people leave you alone. What was once a good boy gone mad, you are going to self-indulge in material objects to fill the void. Being a success in any career path you choose is something that is going to make you flaunt an ego. The jobs are going to give you access to lots of money, and for you with money comes the power. Delusion is going to be your best friend because you are going to feel like money can buy you happiness.

Life is going to prove that theory wrong and you are going to have a lot of traumas to unpack once you receive one of the hardest reality checks.

Little Jamal, you are now a man, but you have no real clue as to what that means. You allowed society to define what it meant to be a man for you, and you will be so far from who God called you to be. You have been living your whole life trying to prove to others that you are worthy to the point it kills you. On the brink of your thirtieth year of life, you get hit with not one, but two strokes. You will suffer with a brain injury for the rest of your life and the Jamal you knew will be erased. You can no longer hide behind your smile and or your fashions ever again. You are going to be forced to deal with all your trauma. Your trauma will be the only remains from your deceased old self. I am sorry, little Jamal, that I treated you so unkind. You were my pride and joy, but I abused you and the world helped me do it. I could've stopped it at any time, but I acted as if I couldn't see it and now you are gone. Being thrust into the medical world as a patient is not what I wanted for you.

I should have encouraged you to keep dreaming, baby, and keep on being beautiful. I was so consumed with making you greater for the next person that I did not invest in you. I didn't protect your heart and I did not protect your mind. I should've trusted God more, but I failed us, Jamal. I wish I could go back and do things over, but I can't, and it hurts me so much. Little Jamal, you've become way too good at goodbyes, and I hate that I had to say goodbye to you. You are me and I'm sorry, I miss you so much. The fact that I hurt you really haunts me; how can I go on? I'm supposed to act like you never existed when you did. There is no grave because you died inside of me, because of you, little Jamal, I walk around with a hole in my heart. I hurt myself by hurting you.

Every day I think of you, little Jamal,. I know you are not coming back, but I decided to honor you through my actions. I speak of you as often as I can, and I share your story because it gives people hope. It makes people aware of your sacrifices and all that you endured. Sharing knowledge about brain injuries makes you relevant and people show appreciation for the enlightenment. Young Jamal, I am now in the fifth year of remission because of God. I just wish you still lived inside of me to celebrate with me. I continue to seek out the help I need to grieve the loss of you in a healthy way and sharing the trauma helps. God is at the beginning and ending of each journey. Our job is just to show up and, little Jamal, that is what I plan to do. I loved you then and now, and I bet I always will.

Manifestation

Since the beginning of all my trauma, I have been speaking out to the universe for better days. I don't know how I knew that things would get better, but I kept fighting for my life, knowing that someday things would. I envisioned my life going forward through the first five as something that would be groundbreaking. I would accomplish several things and I would be the first of many, in which I did! I dreamed during my time of disparity, and in my dream, I would see myself mastering the art of being disabled. I would have premonitions also that one day I would be a source of hope for many people who didn't know me and that included doctors. All these things I thought about and have spoken upon eventually became true. I handled every adversity thrown my way with grace and a lot of people admired my transparency. I had no problem sharing my trials and tribulations with the world, but when it came to my energy I had to think twice.

Everything was going according to my manifestations, and I knew that a part of receiving what I asked for I had to change up my format going forward. Allowing people easy access to me was a struggle for me in my past, and along my spiritual and physical journey I realized I had poor spiritual hygiene. So, it is nothing personal when I state that this Jamal is for me, and you can have my story. I share my highs and lows because character is in there, but I need all my energy for me. Sure, we can match energies if yours is pure, but it is poor spiritual maintenance to deplete myself of energy because I've loaned it all out. I manifested that my sorrow wouldn't be in vain, so I went into every unfortunate situation prepared to win. I spoke victory over my life. Every single one of my wins that people were blessed to see is what I manifested into my life.

I conclude that the old life I was living that caused me to get terribly ill was me having a lack of respect for myself. How dare I abandon my health to a degree that I had headaches daily for ten years. Lesson learned and I vowed to never go back there, so anything that can cause me to lose energy is too expensive for my taste. I said I would shock the world with my inner thoughts and all that I learned from my experience, and just like that, I created my freshmen novel *Master Reset*. That book gained me so much positive notoriety and finally people were paying attention to me for all the right reasons. I exposed the real me, my experience with shady characters, and ultimately my strife with the medical world. God gave me a brain injury and I was going to make the most of my life living with an incurable disease. I didn't ask for it, but I was determined to make something of it. I wanted to show that you could do anything you wanted to do, if you just believe.

I did all that I could to display the light at the end of the tunnel the best way I knew. Sometimes it feels like I am hardly breathing, and I need someone to save me, but I know deep down inside no one is coming because I manifested this aspect as well. I wanted my work to reach the heartstrings of the masses, so even if it seems be a bit much sometimes, I won't complain. People want so much from me at times, and they wish for me to be everywhere at once. It is all about balance, and throughout the first five, I've learned this philosophy and established healthy boundaries. When I speak, people listen and that does magnificent things to my soul because I was the underdog for most of my life. I asked the universe and

God for guidance as to what is next.

I am one of those individuals who paved the way for a lot of young people today. To be yourself was a crime when I was growing up in the late '80s and early '90s. I was one of those kids who would wear my pink and take the beatings afterwards. I just knew in my mind that I was something special, and so my daily affirmation was I am going to be so big that people are going to have to take a number if they would like to hang with me. Fast-forward to now as everyone has come to know, I did not lie. This is my life and I have my friends who are the family I created, and I have my family that I was born into. I truly couldn't ask for a healthier support system. To my supporters I'm thankful that we found each other, and I appreciate you for loving me when you did not have to. For that, I love you all back. I was told I was too much,

I agree with that observation because I am too much. I am real, too transparent, and too blessed. I understand that their feelings of me have nothing to do with me. I am not sure if I hit a nerve in them because they are missing something, and I do not care. I stand and live in my truth, so if I am too much, what you are telling me is that you are simply not enough. I have just begun displaying my light after all I've been through, so if it too bright for you, your best bet would be to purchase some sunglasses. God declared that he wanted me here and God also declared that I am enough, so the opinions of others will never matter. The first five years have been both a physical and emotional fight. I am grateful to still be alive and striving towards my goal. I knew exactly what I would be doing when this year came and that's celebrate my victory. I didn't miss these past five years and that's because of God's mercy, so I plan to show my gratitude.

June 30 is the actual day that will make it five years that I will be in remission. I planned to celebrate that and my thirty-fifth birthday on an all-inclusive vacation. I want to just relax, reflect, and say thank you to the most God for the gift of life again. I now live a life with purpose and life with more accomplishments than I ever saw coming. How I'm living now is the life that I dreamed about, and I am just getting started. I must acknowledge those before me whose shoulders I ride on and all the soldiers that I've lost throughout my first five. They are all missed, and helped shape my idea of helping others because I witnessed too many people leave this world without a village. I've noticed a lack of care for life, and I planned to shed light on that going forward. I pledged to be the change I wished to see and pray others will follow me lead.

I can never forget to speak about my little best friend Azari. This book is dedicated to her. She is my niece, and she was born the year all of this took place five years ago. While I was in and out of the hospital, her little face gave me joy. In my first book, I spoke about how, at times, I felt so lonely (even with family and friends around) suggested that I longed for a lover but in all actuality, I manifested my little best friend. She came into this world right on time and our connection is what I needed. After the doctors told me that I could never have children due to chemo, I just knew I would never know what it would be like to have a little person need me. I just knew I would never get the chance to experience the kind of love I hear parents describe when they speak of their child being born.

I've learned that I don't have to be a dad to receive pure love from a child and my little best friend showed me that, and then some. I love my role as the cool uncle that gives her whatever she desires, and I will always be thankful to her for reminding me that I am wanted. No matter how old she gets, she will always be my beautiful black princess. I needed her more than she will ever know. She allowed me in her world, and she knows she can always count on her uncle Mally. I thought I would never experience this unique bond in my life, so the first five is a celebration of the first five years of my best friend's life and the first five years of me being in remission, and it only gets better from here. Cheers!!!!

www.ingramcontent.com/pod-product-compliance
Lightning Source LLC
LaVergne TN
LVHW010506160826
845677LV00012B/2694